Home Sweet Nursing Home
(Doris)

An A to Z Collection of 50-word stories on aging and healthcare

DORIS PLASTER

Copyright @ 2011 Doris Plaster
All rights Reserved

ISBN:1-4611-1861-1
ISBN-13:978-1-4611-1861-9

Dedication

To Raymond
for his unwavering love and support.

To Ernie
for believing in my dreams ("ay, ño!")

To my friends
for their encouragement.

To my nursing home residents
for enlightening my life all these years.

Doris Plaster

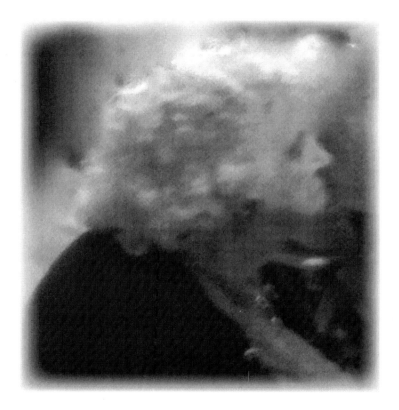

Home Sweet Nursing Home

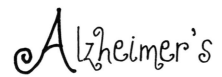

Immersed in her own world, Mrs. Smith wandered the halls of the Alzheimer's unit.

A man and a woman visited her daily. She remained detached, silent.

"It's wonderful that Mrs. Smith has loving visitors, but where's her husband?" a curious nurse asked me.

"That *is* her husband—and his girlfriend."

Doris Plaster

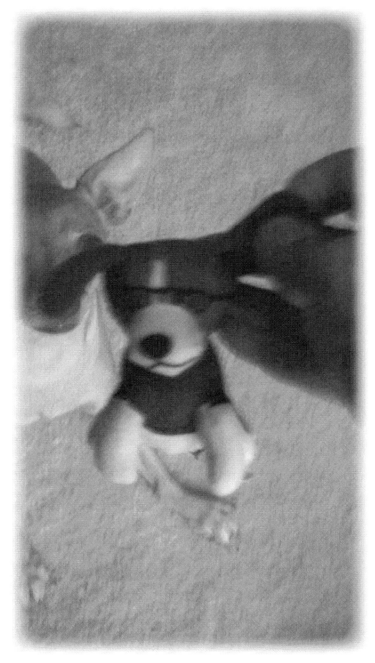

Home Sweet Nursing Home

Bella

Bella was old. She seemed the oldest of all the nursing home occupants.

With a limp, she slowly paced up and down the halls daily.

Some residents would stop to talk to her and pat her on the back.

Bella loved it—then she would beg for her doggie treats.

Doris Plaster

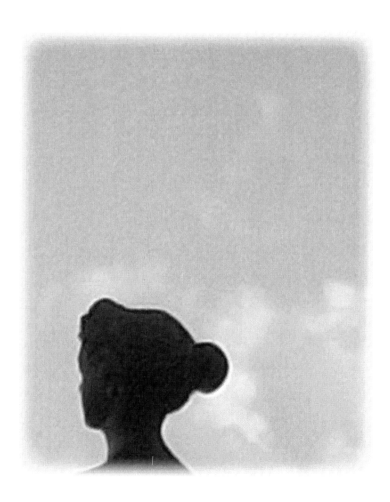

Crystal Clear

"I'm his ex-wife. Why is he in a nursing home?"

"Ma'am, I can't disclose medical information unless his Power of Attorney gives consent," I politely explained.

"His girlfriend is the POA, and she won't."

"I'm sorry."

"F*** you, b****," she screamed and hung up.

Things made perfect sense now.

Doris Plaster

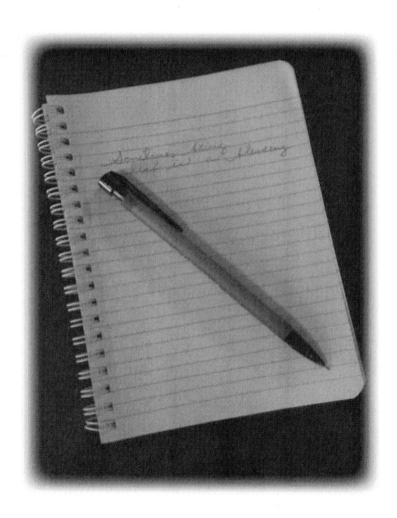

Deafness

Ms. Nolan spied the professionals attending her nursing home care meeting.

Her eyes reflected her clear embarrassment as her daughter spoke in a loud, annoyed manner.

Ms. Nolan was deaf, yet she read lips perfectly.

She reached for her notepad and pen, and wrote:

Sometimes being deaf is a blessing.

Doris Plaster

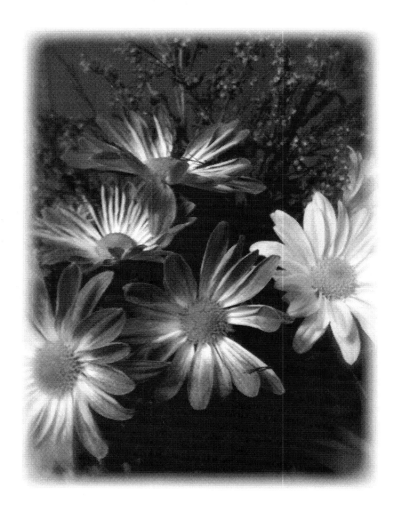

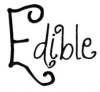

A beautiful daisy plant adorned Ms. Taylor's room.

Her sister, Marilyn, had tried to brighten her day, even if Ms. Taylor was confused and didn't recognize her sister.

"Marilyn, we can't have plants in the dementia unit," a nurse explained. "Residents might eat them."

"Don't worry; the plant isn't poisonous!"

Doris Plaster

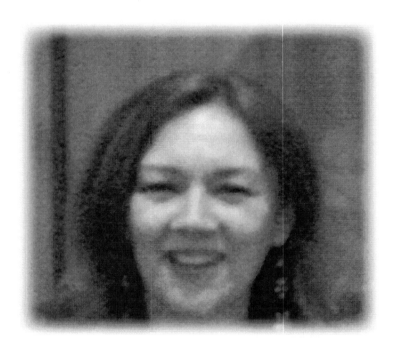

Familiar Face

"Hello!" Ms. Adams greeted everyone who passed by the nurse's desk, her favorite spot and where she perched herself.

"Hi, Ms. Adams," everyone greeted back.

"Hey, you!" She motioned to me. "Do you work here?"

I frowned, sensing her confusion.

"I'm Melba, your social worker."

"Hmm. Your face looks familiar..."

Doris Plaster

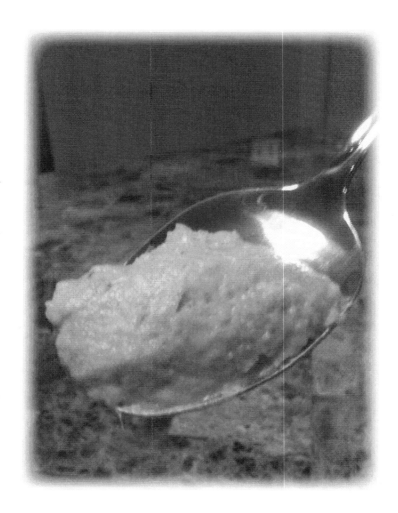

Gourmet

Lunch was served. At times, feeding some of the nursing home residents was a chore.

"Try these delicious peas," I encouraged Ms. Miller, aiming a spoon full of moss-green, gelled, pureed food toward her mouth. "Yummy!"

Ms. Miller gently turned the spoon back to me. "Hon, get you some yourself!"

Doris Plaster

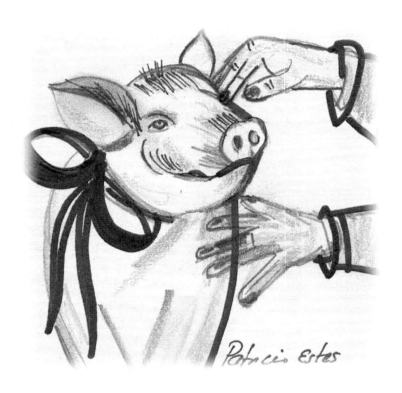

Hallucination

After a week off, Nurse Sylvia returned to the dementia unit.

"Resident exhibits hallucinations. States she was playing with pigs," Sylvia wrote in her nurse's notes.

With her shift over, Sylvia walked down the hall. An old flyer in the trash can caught her attention.

Pet Therapy with Tom's Piggies.

Doris Plaster

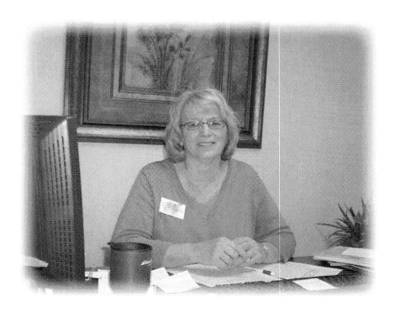

Home Sweet Nursing Home

Imposter

"I'm looking for Cheryl!" Ms. Parker abruptly popped into my office.

"What can I do for you, Ms. Parker?" I smiled.

"You're *not* Cheryl the social worker!" she stammered angrily.

"Ms. Parker, I *am* Cheryl."

"You're dressed like Cheryl, but you are not!"

"Then let me find her for you..."

Doris Plaster

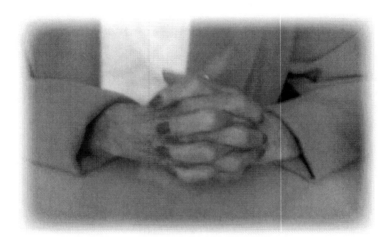

Jeff

"Please, Ms. Schindler, take your pills," a nurse begged.

"Jeff! Jeff! Jeff!" was Ms. Schindler's repetitious reply.

"She's agitated, refusing care, meals—everything!" The nurse grew frustrated.

"Ms. Schindler, Jeff wants you to eat your food and take your medications," I said.

"Huh? He does?" Ms. Schindler's eyes brightened. "Okay."

Doris Plaster

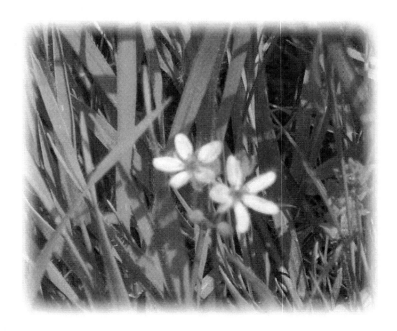

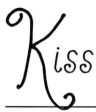iss

"The Alzheimer's unit staff is worried about Ms. Siegel," the activities coordinator reported to me. "She spends the entire day with another resident."

"If they are not harming themselves or others, we should leave them be."

"Well, Ms. Siegel kissed the other resident."

"Who is the other resident?"

"Ms. Brooks."

Doris Plaster

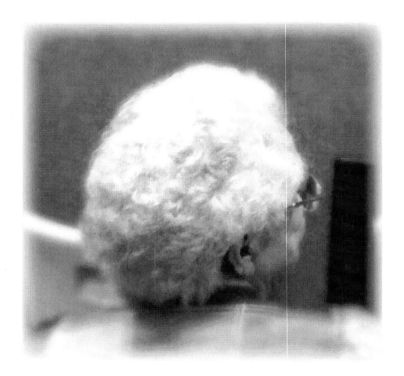

Home Sweet Nursing Home

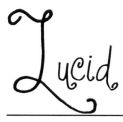

Mother was having a lucid day. But that wasn't usual since she moved into the nursing home.

"I know my mind isn't good. I'm glad you came to see me."

"Mom, you're wonderful. I'll see you next week. I love you."

"Okay, be careful... I love you too, Aunt Julie."

Doris Plaster

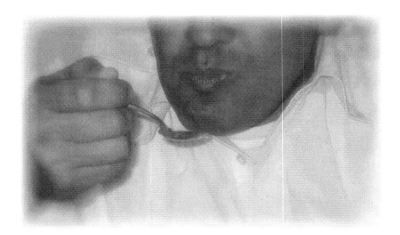

Mental Changes

"My mother's delusional," a distressed woman said, approaching Nurse Margie. "She thinks the staff is eating her meals."

"I'll report this to the attending physician," Margie promised.

Days later, an employee was seen being escorted from the nursing home.

"What happened?" Margie asked.

"He was caught stealing the residents' food."

Doris Plaster

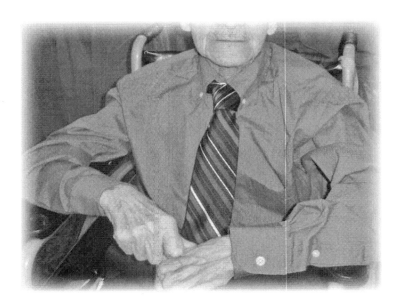

No Doubt

"Mrs. Nicholson, we believe your husband is dying," Nurse Manager Olivia explained.

"I know my husband," Mrs. Nicholson stated. "He will recover."

Two months later, Mr. Nicholson completed rehabilitation successfully.

"Married for sixty-two years." Olivia shook her head. "For Pete's sake, no one knew Mr. Nicholson better than his wife!"

Doris Plaster

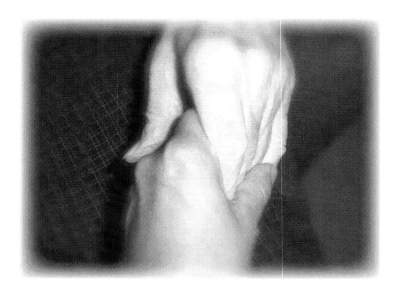

Overstepping Boundaries

Anne held Mr. King's hand. She loved him dearly. Mr. King adored his new girlfriend. They could care less about the gossip about them in the nursing home.

"Why did Anne lose her nursing license?" a curious therapist asked.

"Because she fell for her patient, Mr. King," another therapist whispered.

Doris Plaster

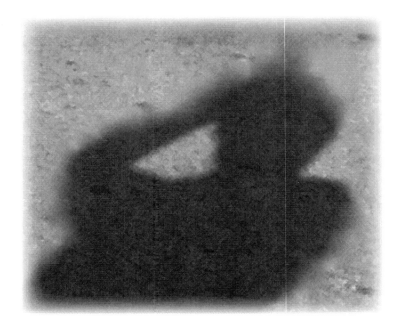

Post-Traumatic Stress Disorder (PTSD)

An agonizing scream echoed down the hall. It was Mr. Colbert's first shower.

"His bath was a battle. He kicked and hit staff," I told his wife.

"Oh, his PTSD! He was a POW—tortured by water immersion."

"Nursing staff to the conference room for in-service," I announced. "Immediately!"

Doris Plaster

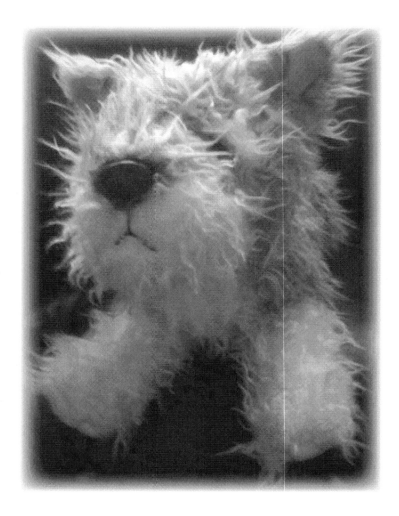

Home Sweet Nursing Home

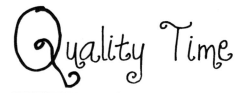

"Boomer! Bad dog!" Ruth yelled. "You know better than to do that!"

Ruth took her loving companion, Boomer, with her everywhere in the nursing home.

Yet she would not tolerate him misbehaving.

Another resident observed the scene. "She and that stuffed animal!" he said, turning back to his Bingo card.

Doris Plaster

Relief

"My daughter is dead! Cindy!" Ms. Grey cried in agony. "It's all over the news!"

Puzzled, I said, "Let's call your family." I punched in Cindy's number nervously.

"Hello?"

"Cindy?"

"Yes."

"Your mother would like to talk with you."

Ms. Grey grabbed the phone. "Cindy, I had a bad dream..."

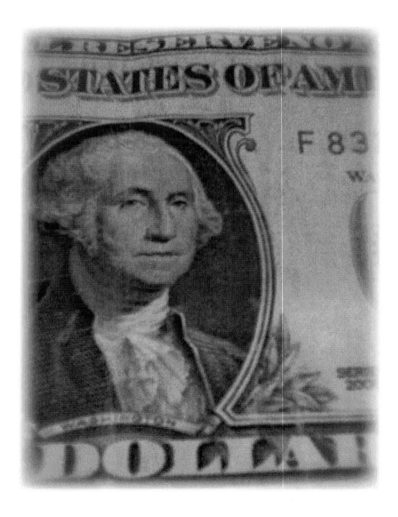

Six-Figure Deal

"I've hired the best attorney in town to represent me in my motor vehicle accident claim," Robert told everyone in the rehabilitation unit. "I'm getting a six-figure deal!"

A year later...

"I saw Robert!" my co-worker exclaimed. "He's homeless. He spent every cent of his hefty settlement in Las Vegas."

Doris Plaster

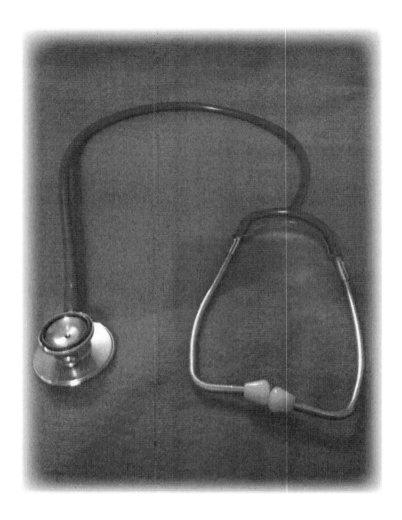

Tough Decisions

"Stop dialysis? No!" Ms. Green's daughter, Kelly, yelled at her sister.

"That's the nephrologist's recommendation," Lucy explained. "Mother's prognosis is poor."

"I'll see you in court!" Kelly exclaimed as she huffed out of the nursing home.

The two sisters never talked again. Not even at Ms. Green's funeral, days later.

Doris Plaster

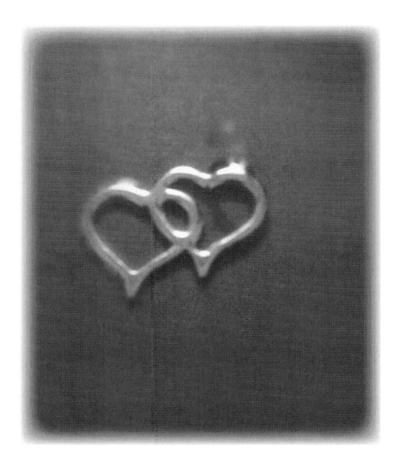

Unfaithfully Faithful

"Why are my husband and that other lady holding hands?" Mrs. Phillips angrily questioned upon entering the Alzheimer's unit.

"I'm sorry, Mrs. Phillips," Nurse Jane said. "We have tried to keep him away from her, but it's almost impossible."

"Why is he after her?"

"Your husband thinks she is *you*."

Doris Plaster

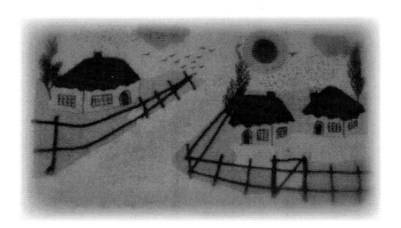

Village

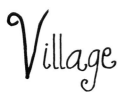

"Ms. Ismail's room is a mess!" a nurse assistant complained. "She's washing her clothes in the trash can and hanging them on the chair backs."

I rushed to her room. A Hindu sign graced her door.

She was diligently folding clothes.

"Visiting my village?" she asked, flashing a charming smile.

Doris Plaster

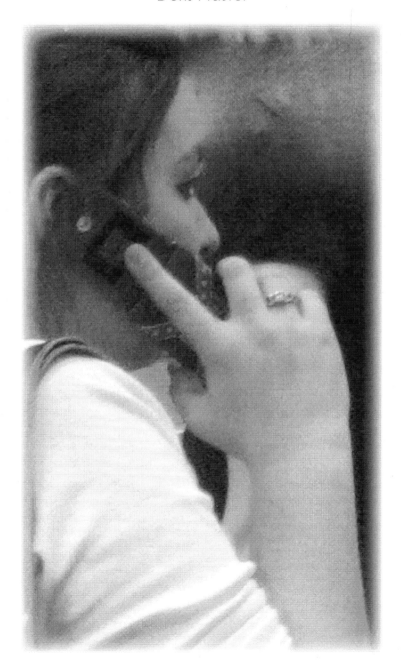

Wrong Number

"What?" Mary gasped for air. "My father's in the ICU?"

"He coded," Nurse Katrina said. "He's unresponsive."

"I'm heading to the hospital right now." Mary hung up. Tears streamed down her cheeks.

The phone rang again.

"Hello?

"Mary, your father's fine," Katrina said. "I'm sorry, I grabbed the wrong chart."

Doris Plaster.

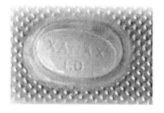
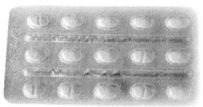

Xanax

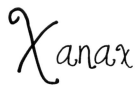

"Allan's visitors are strange people," a nurse commented. "It's rumored they're drug addicts and are stealing Allan's Xanax."

"Nurses dose his Xanax twice a day. There's no way he could pass his pills to his visitors," I assured.

"Except when he spits them out once the nurse leaves the room."

Doris Plaster

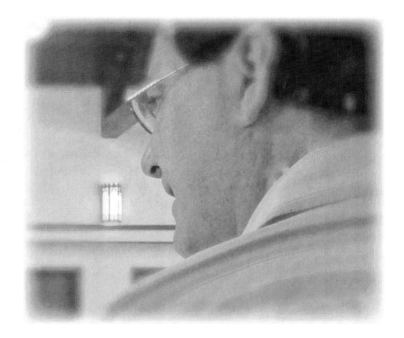

Young Looking

Mrs. Mueller had just arrived at the nursing home. Admission paperwork had to be completed.

Sixty-two-year-old Mrs. Mueller lay in her bed. A thirty-something man sat at her bedside, holding her hand.

"I'm Jerry Mueller. I'll sign her paperwork."

"Good! I'll need your mother's insurance cards."

"She's actually my wife."

Doris Plaster

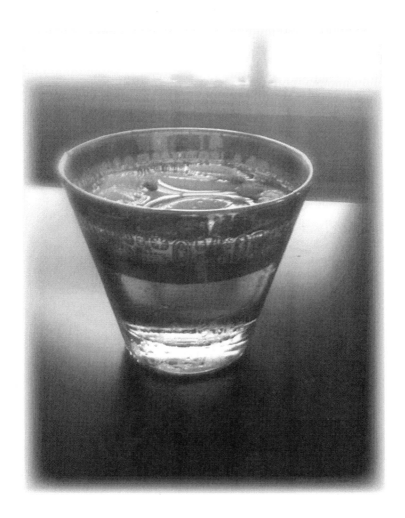

Zestful Patient

Ms. Milton sat before me, asking questions about our nursing home after being referred to me from the hospital's social worker.

"We have private rooms," I explained.

She gazed at me, hesitating.

"Any other questions?"

"What about drinks?"

"We offer juices, tea, coffee..."

"No, I mean, drinks—my evening scotch!"